A Summary of Dr. William Davis' Book:

Wheat Belly

Lose the Wheat, Lose the Weight, and
Find Your Path Back to Health

by Shortcut Summaries

Published by CornerTrade Publishing,
a subsidiary of CornerTrade, LLC

Wheat Belly

Disclaimer

Shortcut Summaries

Contents

Preface

Summary of Dr. William Davis' *Wheat Belly*

While wheat is touted as part of a "heart healthy diet" and we are encouraged to eat more whole grains, the wheat we buy in the supermarket is worlds away, genetically speaking, from the wheat our grandparents ate. Not coincidentally, their generation was far leaner and healthier than ours. Clearly, something radical has changed in our national diet, and the genetic modification of wheat, according to Dr. William Davis MD, is that change. In Section 1, you'll learn just how wheat has changed over the years into the pseudo-food we consume today.

In *Wheat Belly by Dr. William Davis: Lose the Wheat, Lose the Weight and Find Your Path Back to Health,* Dr. Davis makes his case against wheat. Using a combination of his own clinical observations, established medical studies and documented research, Dr. Davis paints a vivid picture of precisely how wheat affects the body. Among other things, it contributes to weight gain, diabetes, heart disease and chronic lethargy. You'll read about the specific effects on each body system in Section 2.

Going wheat-free can seem intimidating or impossible, given how much wheat we actually eat on a regular basis. However, in Section 3, you'll learn the fundamentals of eliminating wheat and, better still, how to replace it with foods you'll actually enjoy eating!

Wheat Belly Section 1a

Wheat Isn't Wheat Anymore

As a society, we are fat. This is a fact acknowledged by every medical organization, and can easily be verified by a quick glance at your friends, family and neighbors. Many of them probably sport beer bellies, big thighs or the dreaded man-breasts.

Why we're fat, and getting fatter, has baffled dieters for years. According to government medical agencies, it's because we overeat, we're sedentary and load up on junk instead of healthy food. While these things are likely contributors, Dr. Davis maintains they are not the reason we're fat.

The reason is wheat. It sounds almost sacrilege to paint wheat as the bad guy. Since Biblical times, bread and wheat have symbolized wholesome nourishment.

What's key, however, is that the bread broken at the Last Supper – and at your grandparents' dinner table – was an entirely different substance than what's now available in supermarkets. Dr. Davis likens the comparison of old wheat and modern wheat to the comparison of chimps and humans. We might share 99% of our DNA with chimps, but that one percent makes a massive difference.

Surprising Results

After first experimenting with a wheat-free diet himself and then prescribing that diet to his patients, Dr. Davis has come to believe that modern wheat, more than any other grain, is responsible for our societal weight gain. After eliminating wheat, Dr. Davis' patients lost weight easily, reported highly unexpected clearings of chronic diseases and conditions, and felt more alert and energetic.

A Widespread and Familiar Enemy

Wheat is singled out for two main reasons. It has been genetically modified more than other grains such as spelt or barley. In addition, a truly huge portion of our diets contain wheat. We were raised on it and we've raised our children on it, believing it to be healthy. Once upon a time, it was.

Wheat is one of the most widely consumed foods on the planet, accounting for approximately 20% of our overall caloric intake. It is in nearly everything most of us eat, at every meal and every snack.

What Happened?

Due to wheat's huge popularity, it is commercially farmed. This is where the change began.

Crops have long been modified to make them more resistant to insects, fungi and other profit-draining occurrences. Wheat, being the chief profit crop for much of the world, has undergone more modification than any other substance. It has been cross-bred and hybridized.

The biggest goal, even more than resistance to external elements, has been creating wheat which yields the biggest harvest possible. This is why current commercial wheat crops grow to only eighteen inches in height. Profits from these modifications are high, but as Dr. Davis illustrates, they've come at a heavy price.

Consider sheer numbers. Wheat can trace its ancestry back to a handful of strains of wild grain picked by our ancient ancestors. Today, there are over 25,000 strains, nearly all resulting from human modification. Nearly all of this modification occurred after 1950, meaning that the flour used by our grandparents was, for all intents and purposes, the same as flour ground by primitive tools in prior centuries.

While today's wheat may taste and look the same, the differences are crucial. Hybridization and modification have resulted in minute differences in the plant's protein structure. Unfortunately for us, these subtle changes can mean the difference between a healthy, wholesome food and a trigger for systemic changes which initiate a vast range of chronic diseases.

Old-School Wheat

In the beginning, there was einkorn. This ancient grain is like the godfather to all of today's wheat strains, and was eaten by people in Europe as early as 3300 BC. In the Middle East, a variety known as emmer emerged, the result of a natural "mating" between einkorn and wild grass. Emmer was preferable for grinding and cooking, and became predominant for centuries.

At some unclear point which predates Biblical times, emmer grass mated again, with another wild grass species. This union resulted in what was, up until approximately fifty years ago, commonly recognized wheat.

When plants mate, they combine their genetic codes. In humans, our parents' respective 46 chromosomes do not combine into offspring with 92 chromosomes; they are blended so we each have our own set of forty-six. Plants aren't quite as complex, and simply lump their chromosomes together.

Einkorn has 14 chromosomes, emmer wheat 28 courtesy of its goat-grass genes. After its last major mating, wheat ended up with 42 chromosomes. Why is this important? It gave future scientists and geneticists plenty to work with when they began altering wheat to increase resistance and yield.

Preserving the Past

So whatever happened to einkorn and emmer wheat? They did survive, but just barely. Today, they are being cultivated with renewed interest by a handful of dedicated farmers. These small-scale operations rely on ancient and organic methods, producing grains which are virtually identical to what our ancestors ate.

Taste is reported to be much more appealing, and these grains are suggested to be free of virtually all of modern wheat's disease-causing effects.

Today's Franken-Food

Thousands of genetic manipulations separate today's wheat from its ancestors. We have created strains so unnatural that they literally can't survive without human intervention and maintenance.

Some of these genetic strains are designed to work well with certain fertilizers and pesticides. These are many of the highest-profit strains and tend to be dominant in our diets.

In Wheat Belly, Dr. Davis asks the reader to consider the bizarre quality of this manual interference in nature – would we purposely create an animal which would die without a highly specialized diet, available only through humans? The idea is almost offensive, but it's precisely what we've done in the world of agriculture.

Good Intentions

Dwarf or semi-dwarf wheat accounts for approximately ninety percent of the world's wheat crops. These tiny strains were created to increase yield, with the noble intention of producing more disease-resistant and durable wheat to feed starving nations. Species were bred with their parents and other "related" strains to achieve short stalks, which don't break under the heavy load of their huge (thanks to heavy nitrogen fertilizing) seed head.

While the experiments achieved their goals, the results came at a price.

Lack of Forethought

The scientists who produced dwarf wheat strains had a wonderful goal, but didn't think about the potential ramifications of what they were doing. Nobody thought to research or test the effects of genetically modified food. The resulting products would still be "wheat," it was believed, and so would be as well-tolerated as the strains with which the scientists had begun tinkering.

This lack of testing may have been a dire mistake. Modern testing shows that gluten, the primary "ingredient" in wheat which our bodies react to, is highly increased in modern, modified strains. Hybridization produces new proteins, brand-new molecules which neither parent plant contained. In addition, genes responsible for gluten are increased.

Clearly, the wheat we consume today is not, as many scientists would have you believe, the same wheat our ancestors relied upon. It doesn't taste or look the same and, most importantly, it does not have the same effects on our bodies.

Dr. Davis conducted an experiment on himself, using einkorn grain obtained from a small, organic farmer and the same amount of modern, organic whole wheat flour. With his wheat sensitivity, Dr. Davis became nauseated and had trouble concentrating after just four ounces of bread made with modern wheat.

Einkorn flour, interestingly, yielded no such side effects and left the doctor feeling perfectly normal. Not a formally documented scientific experiment, but highly interesting.

Things are poised to get even more complicated as

the field of genetics surges forward. Instead of the old methods, scientists can now remove a single gene from one plant and insert it in another, much the same way would-be parents can choose their future baby's eye color.

All of this was seen as benign until very recently, when the effects of genetically modified foods began to be tested. One disturbing case showed that cattle fed a modified strain of soybeans (created specifically to resist a harsh chemical pesticide) showed changes in their intestinal, liver, pancreatic and testicular tissues.

No such testing was required or even conceived of years ago, when most of today's wheat strains were created. Genetic modifying and hybridization has the power to turn on or off certain genes in wheat. What these genes do when we ingest them is, presently, unknown, and the number of such modifications is impossible to estimate.

Despite all the testing required today, most of the wheat we are eating got into our food supply with no testing, speculation or even thought as to what these modified strains might do to the human body.

Understanding Your Food – A Breakdown of Wheat

Seventy-five percent of the complex carbohydrates in

wheat are amylopectin, branching chains of glucose which our bodies readily convert into sugar. While these chains are certainly found in other foods, wheat contains the type of amylopectin most readily converted into sugar, thus delivering the highest blood-sugar spike.

These compounds (properly called amylopectin A) raise blood sugar even higher and faster than the much-vilified simple sugars we've all been warned for years to avoid. In the simplest terms, the so-called "healthy complex carbs" of modern wheat are worse for blood sugar levels than almost any other type of sugar or carbohydrate.

For a real-world example, Dr. Davis offers the reality that consuming two slices of whole-wheat bread is the same, in terms of increased blood sugar, as drinking a can of sugary soda.

This translates very simply into weight gain and diabetic issues. Our modern wheat raises and sustains blood sugar faster and higher than any other carb. Sugars trigger the release of insulin. Excess insulin causes the body to store fat in its cells, rather than burning it up for energy.

Even more disturbing, the two types of fat (based on body location) most commonly associated with increased insulin levels are belly and organ deposits. These fats are among the most dangerous when it comes to mortality and chronic disease.

The cycle perpetuates itself because the fats within these deposits are usually insulin resistant, meaning that more insulin is needed to trigger their release. The larger these fat deposits become, the more they trigger the body's inflammatory response, which, in turn, triggers chronic disease such as cancer.

Furthering the cycle, wheat stimulates the appetite, inducing cravings for – surprise, surprise – more carbs such as wheat. Wheat also affects the brain in a manner not unlike morphine, making us happy, although that happiness is followed by a familiar, hungry crash.

Eliminating wheat products breaks this cycle, allowing the body to burn its fat stores. In numerous studies, patients dropped amazing amounts of weight on a wheat-free diet.

Despite the scientific evidence showing precisely what wheat does in the body, these studies are often interpreted as working because of a lack of variety in the diet. In other words, scientists say that subjects lose weight because they're bored with their limited choices, when in fact they are free to eat many formerly "forbidden" foods such as cheese, eggs and red meat.

Popular medical advice tells us to eat more complex

carbs. An extremely popular suggestion is whole wheat. The complex carbs in modern whole wheat, however, are actually worse for weight gain, diabetes and many other diseases than dumping spoonfuls of sugar into your morning coffee (not that that's a good idea either).

A Disturbing Alliance?

Dr. Davis points out that highly modified wheat, and modified crops in general, are highly profitable. They often work with a single fertilizer – often a brand-name, patented fertilizer – in order to survive pest attacks.

Some think it disturbing that the type of crops which are pushed by mainstream medical advice are the same ones which yield the highest profits for a variety of Big Business industries, including, pesticide and pharmaceutical companies.

What's the Deal with Gluten?

We hear a lot about gluten these days. More foods than ever are showing up in gluten-free varieties, the option is becoming as popular as vegetarian when choosing meal options at a wedding reception, and entire restaurants and even bakeries are devoted to a life free of gluten. Just what is this mysterious and often highly allergic substance?

Gluten is responsible for most of the qualities we

associate with wheat, such as the stretchiness of dough and how it rises. Other flours, such as those made from rice or corn, can't do what wheat flour can; they crumble under many cooking methods which modern wheat adapts to readily. Note that ancient forms of wheat also tend to crumble.

Modern wheat is only 10% to 15% protein, but up to 80% of the protein in wheat is gluten. Since gluten gives wheat its versatile baking possibilities, geneticists have produced strains with much higher levels of gluten than were ever present in nature, thereby raising the very substance which triggers such a negative allergic response in sensitive individuals and those with celiac disease.

Beyond Gluten

There is more to wheat than this substance, including a host of proteins, carbohydrates and other compounds which are present in modern wheat in much higher levels and genetically different forms than old-school wheat. Human response to these substances is varied; some people react violently while others show no immediate effects whatsoever.

The fact remains, however, that we simply don't yet know what these engineered substances are doing to our bodies, and what little we do know doesn't look good.

Key Points of Wheat Belly Section 1a

Today's wheat is fundamentally different from the wheat we ate just two generations ago.

Genetic modification and hybridization have resulted in wheat with innumerable genetic differences. The effects of these modified genes are largely unknown.

Genetically modified crops have been shown to negatively affect livestock.

While we are told that whole grains are part of a healthy diet, they behave in the body harmfully as simple sugars, quickly raising blood sugar and insulin levels, storing excess fat and eventually causing or contributing to virtually all chronic disease.

Going wheat-free has been shown to have hugely beneficial results on health and obesity, yet these studies are largely ignored by popular medicine.

Modern wheat has been engineered to contain substantially more allergy-provoking proteins than its more natural ancestors.

Nearly all of the modified wheat we consume was introduced long before testing of modified crops was required.

In addition to being modified to increase gluten, many companies add enzymes to flour to increase its baking versatility. Soy flour is another common additive. As a result, today's wheat products contain many untested and unique compounds not found anywhere else, compounds that would not exist without human intervention.

Wheat Belly: Section 1b

Wheat's Effects on Your Belly, Brain and Gut

While some people scoff at the idea of any food – especially something as seemingly innocuous as wheat – being addictive, the evidence points in a different direction. For years, people have reported symptoms such as cravings, dreaming about their "food of choice," lethargy, nervousness and an inability to control their wheat cravings.

Conversely, when they give in to their cravings, they feel something akin to euphoria, leading to them to consume more wheat products. Their particular trigger can be any wheat-based food, but when you take away the product itself, these symptoms sound suspiciously like addiction to any drug.

It is also worth noting that those who stop eating wheat products often say that they are less moody, can think more clearly and have increased energy.

Why does wheat affect us this way? The first studies on wheat and the mind took place during the 1960s. Schizophrenic patients were given a diet free of wheat products, without their knowledge. While there were no miraculous recoveries, nearly all subjects showed a marked improvement in symptoms. When wheat was re-introduced to their diet, their symptoms returned.

One particularly startling case did actually show a "cure," although this is a single incidence and must be considered as such. Dr. Davis finds it unlikely that wheat actually caused schizophrenia in these patients, although the worsening of symptoms can't be ignored.

Studies on autism and ADHD have shown remarkably similar correlations due to wheat in the diet.

What Wheat Does in Your Mind

As your body is digesting wheat, the gluten in wheat itself is broken down into many different compounds, one of which is a particular set of polypeptides. These polypeptides have the unique ability to penetrate the membrane which separates the brain from the blood.

Certain compounds in different things we eat affect

the brain, and so this membrane exists to help keep us in balance. Digested wheat can easily penetrate this membrane, and when it does, it goes straight for our morphine receptor. This is the very same area of the brain targeted by opiate drugs, including heroin.

A group of scientists called these polypeptides "exorphins." You've probably heard of endorphins – the body's natural-high chemicals created by a hard workout. Exorphins are similar compounds created by an external stimulus.

When an individual addicted to heroin is brought into a hospital or detox center, they are often given a drug called naloxone. This drug blocks the effects of heroin, essentially turning a strung-out addict sober in a matter of minutes. This very same drug blocks the effects of wheat on the brain.

Wheat also has the unique ability (among natural foods) to increase the appetite. After removing wheat from their diets, numerous patients have reported a decrease or elimination of their cravings, cravings which previously seemed too strong to resist.

Wheat and Big Business

Whether on purpose or not, the current obesity epidemic started in the 1960s as medical professionals scrambled for a cure for heart disease, cancer, and other chronic diseases. It was discovered that when white flour was replaced with whole wheat flour, cancer rates dropped. Authorities followed the logic that if whole wheat could lower risk, eating a great deal of whole wheat must, therefore, be extremely healthy.

Keep in mind that this is the time period during which hybridization really took off, allowing large food manufacturers to fit their objectives neatly within the medical objectives being put forth by the government – eat more whole grains and be healthier!

Whether the enormous profits created by this comfortable association – a nation addicted to foods which make them want to eat more of those foods, a nation of overweight individuals with chronic diseases which create billions of dollars in revenue for medical and pharmaceutical companies, a nation believing that they're "eating healthy" by ingesting the very things which are making them sick and fat – were known at the time is mere speculation. However, the results are impossible to ignore.

Wheat and Internal Organ Fat

Wheat is also unique in its ability to create and sustain fat around our internal organs (called visceral fat), including the intestines, kidneys, liver, pancreas and even the heart. Wheat is also exceptional at producing this same type of fat around the midsection, for reasons which continue to elude medical science.

Belly fat is deadly in a way that other types of fat are not. Fat in this area of the body triggers the body's inflammatory response, which floods the body with chemicals contributing to a host of chronic diseases. Worse, one of the effects of belly fat is a craving for more food, specifically wheat products.

Wheat is so harmful because of its effects on blood sugar. Wheat is converted to sugar, which triggers the pancreas to produce insulin. Higher levels of sugar produce higher levels of insulin, which trigger the storage of fat, rather than the burning of that fat for energy. This cycle is difficult to break and can very quickly lead to high blood sugar, obesity and diabetes.

It is worth noting that whole wheat bread actually has a higher glycemic index than table sugar.

Wheat and Man-Breasts

Whether you have them, dread them or find them morbidly fascinating, man-breasts are a very real phenomenon. With the exception of cases in which a true hormone imbalance is to blame, many of the man-breasts you see on the street can be traced back to wheat.

Belly fat is a production ground for estrogen. In women this is not as big a deal (although still unhealthy in unnatural levels), but for men it's downright humiliating. Increased estrogen stimulates men to grow breast tissue.

Celiac Disease Data Twisting

Celiac disease, a medically recognized sensitivity to gluten, has been researched for many years. Restricting all wheat products from the diet of an emaciated celiac sufferer nearly always leads to weight gain, simply because their healed systems are able to properly digest food.

However, more recently, overweight individuals have begun showing up in doctors' offices with celiac disease. In these patients, removing wheat gluten caused weight loss, not gain. These studies are documented thoroughly, yet many experts refuse to acknowledge the remarkable correlation.

Dr. Davis looks at the evidence in a different way, asserting that removing wheat, even from the diet of overweight individuals without celiac disease, is a simple, drug-free and surgery-free method of weight loss. Yet this idea is blatantly ignored by mainstream medical society.

Dramatic and Rapid Weight Loss

Over and over, Dr. Davis has seen patients drop as much as ten pounds in two weeks simply by removing wheat from their diets – no other restrictions were in place. How is it possible to lose the same amount of weight, while eating things like steak with blue cheese, as patients on a foodless fast?

Dr. Davis suspects that the reason lies in the interruption of the glucose-insulin-fat-storage connection. He also suspects that once wheat and its accompanying cravings are removed, overall caloric intake goes down naturally.

Skipping Gluten-Free Foods

In large part as a response to those with celiac disease, a host of gluten-free foods have appeared on store shelves. They sound good, but they're typically made with rice, corn, and potato or tapioca starches. Instead of being healthy, these products are actually among the very few which increase blood glucose faster and higher than wheat! Instead of eating these fake foods, in Wheat Belly, Dr. Davis recommends eating a diet rich in naturally gluten-free foods versus fabricated ones.

A Closer Look at Celiac Disease

Celiac disease is intolerance to wheat gluten. Like the also-familiar lactose intolerance, it represents a portion of society which has not yet become used to a new food group. Dr. Davis is quick to point out that his book is not about celiac disease, but it bears mention simply because it is not unlike a measuring stick for all other forms of wheat intolerance.

A typical celiac sufferer endures pain, diarrhea and a

host of other ailments after even the tiniest amount of wheat. While once rather rare, it is on the rise, which Dr. Davis attributes to the drastic changes wheat itself has undergone.

The lining of a celiac sufferer's intestines breaks down upon exposure to wheat gluten, leading to severe digestive upset, an inability to absorb key nutrients, internal bleeding and the introduction of substances into the body which are naturally intended to remain in the intestines.

The introduction of these substances into the rest of the body is responsible for an amazing variety of wheat-related disorders. Emotional and mental illness, skin rashes, liver disease, diabetes, autoimmune diseases, neurological conditions and severe nutritional deficiencies are just a few of the issues created by specific wheat substances perforating the intestinal lining.

Interestingly, several studies have shown that modern wheat, compared with relatively "pure" strains from years ago, triggers celiac disease and other, less severe wheat sensitivities in much higher levels. Something we've done to wheat is obviously having very serious consequences.

It's important to remember that many wheat-triggered disorders and symptoms can show up and wreak havoc in patients who test negative for celiac disease.

If you are experiencing these symptoms, Dr. Davis suggests a wheat-elimination trial.

Wheat, one of our most beloved foods, actually has a mortality rate. In a study covering people with wheat sensitivity (not just celiac disease) increased mortality rates jumped nearly 30%, compared with wheat-neutral individuals. It is interesting that a food which our government encourages us to eat on a daily basis has its very own mortality rate.

Acid Reflux and IBS

Although not usually associated with celiac disease or wheat intolerance in general, acid reflux and irritable bowel syndrome have both shown marked improvement on a wheat-free diet.

Key Points of Wheat Belly Section 1b

Wheat shows the very same addictive properties as illicit drugs, including cravings and withdrawal.

Wheat elimination reduced schizophrenic symptoms in psychiatric patients.

Wheat affects the same area of the brain as heroin or morphine.

Drugs which block the "high" of heroin also block the effects of addictive wheat behavior.

Wheat is an appetite stimulant.

Understanding how wheat works in the body gives us an excellent basis for losing weight through eliminating wheat.

Wheat creates belly and visceral fat, which stimulates the blood sugar-glucose-insulin response. A big belly is essentially a factory for chemicals which make and keep us sick and fat.

Belly fat from wheat consumption stimulates estrogen production, creating man-breasts.

Is there a correlation between big farming, big business and big pharmaceuticals, since all these corporate giants have a vested interested in promoting wheat and then treating the conditions which wheat creates?

"Gluten-free" foods are typically unhealthy due to high glycemic additives.

Wheat elimination generally results in weight loss (for the overweight) even in those who show no obvious symptoms of wheat sensitivity.

Celiac disease is on the rise, along with IBS and acid reflux. Numbers started rising at approximately the same time genetically modified wheat became commonplace.

Wheat Belly: Section 2

Wheat's Effects on Diabetes, pH and Aging

Not surprisingly, given its effects on blood sugar, Dr. Davis asserts that wheat is a fast-track to diabetes. By removing wheat from your diet, a host of conditions would go along with it, including overeating, visceral fat, insulin resistance, high blood sugar, the body's inflammatory response, glycation, triglycerides and small, dense LDL cholesterol.

In the 1920s when insulin therapy was discovered, many childhood diabetic lives were saved. Nobody noticed, however, that adults didn't need more insulin – they were already making too much! This was discovered in the 1950s, followed by the discovery of insulin resistance in the 1980s.

Insulin resistance research led to the now-familiar admonitions to eat more "healthy whole grains," which has since its inception, led to a nation of overweight and diabetic individuals. The incidence of diabetes in adults, in fact, remained fairly steady until the mid-1980s, when major medical associations began to recommend more grains – then, it shot up to levels never seen before.

Even worse, studies show us that for each diabetic, there are at least three people with pre-diabetes, a collection of symptoms including impaired glucose tolerance, high blood sugar and metabolic syndrome. Still, we are told to eat more whole grains.

Wheat and Your Pancreas

On average, a person today eats twenty-six pounds more wheat per year than in 1970. In addition to the aforementioned consequences, all that wheat takes its toll on the pancreas. Pancreatic beta cells are responsible for creating insulin. As our bodies become pre-diabetic, up to 50 percent more of these cells are created to keep up with the demand for insulin created by increased blood sugar levels.

Pancreatic beta cells are actually damaged, however, by glucotoxicity (essentially high blood sugar) and by lipotoxicity (high levels of triglycerides and fatty acids in the blood). Other pre-diabetic conditions can kill off these beta cells, eventually reducing them to approximately fifty percent of their initial number. Once this level is reached, a person is considered irreversibly diabetic since their pancreas simply can't keep up with their blood glucose levels.

Wheat and the ADA (American Diabetes Association)

Currently, the prescribed diet for a diabetic includes large portions of wheat products on a daily basis. In essence, they are telling diabetics to eat more of what is making them sick, ignoring evidence which points to a cure.

Dr. Davis asserts that by following a reduced or wheat-free diet, many diabetics could essentially be cured. Not just managed, but cured. This opinion (and the science backing it up) is not new, yet it continues to be ignored by the largest medical association that focuses on diabetes.

Childhood diabetes, which is on the rise, may also be linked to exposure to today's mutated wheat while in the womb. More studies are needed to confirm this.

Wheat and Your Body's pH Levels

The body has a strict acid/alkaline level it must maintain in order to survive. This level is so important that the body will readily draw calcium from bones in order to maintain balance. The bulk of the acid in our diet typically comes from animal-based foods. These foods, however, also have certain properties which help prevent them from throwing our pH balance out of whack. Plant-based foods give us our alkaline sources.

Grains are unique among plant foods in that they generate acidic by-products, wheat being one of the worst offenders. Since we eat far more wheat than any other grain, wheat can be thanked for much of the prevalence and early onset of osteoporosis we are seeing in our society.

The more wheat we eat (which does not have the built-in safety measures of animal-based foods), the more our bones are depleted to keep pH in check. Soon, mineral loss, osteoporosis and fractures follow.

Wheat and Aging

Wheat contributes to both visible and invisible signs of aging in a variety of ways. Arthritis, considered a disease of older individuals, is made worse by wheat induced belly fat, since this unique type of fat contributes to inflammation which, in turn, contributes to the breakdown of joint cartilage.

Glycation also plays a role in joint destruction. Since all joints are affected, this explains why the hands of an overweight person are as affected by arthritis as the knees, even though the hands don't carry excess weight.

Dr. Davis relates one startling case in which one of his patients, a man nearly crippled by joint pain, was able to walk freely with no pain after three months on a wheat-free diet.

Diabetes has given medical science a perfect method for studying the effects of accelerated aging. Several conditions, including stroke, high blood pressure and cancer, among others, are present in diabetics long before they appear in a normal, healthy individual.

Essentially, this shows us that anything which drives up blood glucose also accelerates the aging process.

Advanced glycation end-products (AGEs) are a rather recent but hugely important discovery when it comes to how and why we age. These compounds can enter the body as part of foods we eat, but are also the waste products of glycation, a process driven by high blood sugar. AGEs accumulate wherever they are created, sitting around doing nothing of value.

They form cataracts, stiffen arteries and cloud neuron communication in the brain, creating dementia. They accumulate in virtually every organ, slowing the function of that organ. They even collect in the skin, leading to visible wrinkles. In effect, AGEs are the waste products of metabolic syndrome and one of (if not the) leading cause of premature aging.

In the blood, diabetics have a much higher level of AGEs than non-diabetics, showing the link between this disease, its many debilitating counterparts and the accelerated aging process.

Kidney disease, Alzheimer's, heart disease, erectile dysfunction, eye health and even cancer have all been linked to AGE accumulation. They do a lot of their damage through oxidation and inflammation, two processes linked to most of the chronic, progressive conditions already linked to being overweight and having diabetes.

Wheat products, more than almost every other food, create more AGEs faster upon consumption, thanks to their quickly processed amylopectin, resulting in rapid blood sugar levels.

Dr. Davis notes that fructose, especially high-fructose corn syrup, produces hundreds of times more AGEs than glucose.

Some AGEs are consumed instead of created, and they are mostly found in meats. In order to cut down on ingesting AGEs, Dr. Davis suggests avoiding cured meats and foods which have been deep-fried or cooked at high temperatures for long periods of time.

With all the available science, something is becoming clear – eating wheat-free is not only beneficial to your current health, but may very well be the anti-aging breakthrough so many have been searching for.

Size Matters

Large and small LDL (low-density lipoprotein) particles play a crucial role in heart disease, although they are poorly understood by most doctors. The larger your LDL particles, the less likely they are to accumulate in arteries. Therefore, smaller LDL particles put you at a greater risk for heart disease and stroke.

Cholesterol measuring is outdated, from a time when today's advanced identification of HDL, LDL, small and large LDL and a host of other minute differences simply were not possible to measure. Doctors cling to measuring cholesterol, sadly, because it's easy and inexpensive.

Large LDL particles are recognized and processed normally by the liver, while small LDL particles are not, giving them more time in the bloodstream to do their damage. In addition, oxidation and glycation occurs more readily in small LDL particles and, in turn, oxidized and glycated LDL particles are more harmful.

A single item fuels all this extremely efficiently; carbohydrates, the chief of which is wheat. Wheat creates more small LDL particles, contributes to their oxidization and glycation. Wheat also contributes to inflammation and a host of other chronic-disease-causing conditions. Removing wheat from the diet not only drastically reduces the levels of small LDL particles, but eases these other conditions as well.

Current popular methods of testing LDL levels do not actually measure LDL levels, don't take into account the size of the LDL particles and are highly flawed, with many factors capable of throwing off the results. In spite of this, statin drugs are prescribed with unswerving regularity, based on these faulty tests.

Because fats contain triglycerides, they have been

thought of as evil, driving up our cholesterol/triglyceride levels. In reality, studies have proven that fat has little to no overall effect on triglyceride levels. Carbs, however, stimulate insulin production, which triggers the liver to release triglycerides. Eating a "heart healthy" diet that promotes the consumption of grains like wheat can actually create fatty liver disease and liver cirrhosis in non-alcoholics.

A host of other heart-disease-triggering conditions are created by eating a diet high in carbs, and most of us get a huge percentage of our carbs from wheat. By eliminating wheat, Dr. Davis claims it is possible to reverse or at least stop the progress of these conditions, often achieving the desired (but rarely achieved) results of prescription medications without the cost or side effects of these drugs.

Wheat and Your Brain

Overeating due to increased hunger is an obvious behavioral effect of wheat. However, there are physical effects that are more "hidden" and take place deep within the brain. Unfortunately, these effects can be life-altering and often can't be reversed.

One example is ataxia. This paralyzing disorder is often seen in celiac sufferers. However, many patients show no symptoms for the wheat allergies which we associate with celiac disease. Symptoms include balance issues and stumbling and often progress to incontinence. There is no known cause or cure, but blood analysis often shows abnormal gluten blood markers.

A host of neurological issues can stem from undiagnosed wheat sensitivity because the inflammatory response which celiac sufferers experience in their digestion can also target virtually any area of the body. When it targets the brain, neurological symptoms appear, often baffling doctors.

Dr. Davis suggests a wheat-free trial for anybody with unexplained neurological issues, including balance or pain. His case studies include a woman who could barely stand due to foot pain who, after two wheat-free weeks, was virtually pain free.

Currently the full extent of wheat's potential effects on the brain is unknown; more research is needed. Seizures are a potential symptom. While gluten is often the culprit, other wheat side-effects can harm the brain and the two groups of effects (gluten and non-gluten) feed off of and worsen each other.

Wheat and Your Skin

Skin is the body's largest organ, and just as susceptible to wheat damage as any other. Wrinkles and aging are just some of the signs, but there are many others.

Acne is a great example simply because it's so

prevalent. Interestingly, many cultures around the world experience virtually no acne whatsoever. The majority of these cultures also consume little to no sugars, wheat or dairy products. In several cases, when a Westernized diet was introduced to such cultures, acne showed up soon after (along with a host of serious chronic diseases).

While a dietary explanation for acne has been dismissed for years, recent studies are pointing at insulin as a very real cause. This brings acne research full-circle, since early in the 20th century acne was commonly blamed on starches. Current studies are proving this old-school wisdom correct, with wheat-restricted test subjects showing as much as a 50% reduction in acne flares.

Dermatitis herpetiformis (DH) is another way wheat can manifest on the skin. This disorder is not a form of herpes; it simply mimics that virus' appearance in some cases. DH can show up anywhere on the body and requires thorough testing for diagnosis. People with DH often show the same intestinal damage as celiac sufferers, but do not actually suffer the same symptoms. DH is often treated with a highly toxic medication with frightening side effects, while wheat elimination can accomplish the same results.

Other topical conditions linked to wheat consumption include ulcers in the mouth, psoriasis, Vitiligo and Behcet's disease.

This is just a small sampling of a frightening list, potentially leading to permanent scarring and even amputation. Worse yet, it's an incomplete list. Wheat can affect the skin in many other ways as well. A particularly visible one is hair loss, occasionally the whole-body hair loss known as alopecia.

No other food has been linked to as many potential skin issues as wheat. Before smearing on a potent, painful cream that turns you into a sun-fearing vampire, consider wheat sensitivity. The solution may be as simple as eliminating this multi-tasking threat from your diet.

Key Points of Wheat Belly Section 2

Wheat contributes to many factors of diabetes and metabolic syndrome including increased appetite, visceral fat, insulin resistance, high blood sugar, inflammation, Glycation, LDL cholesterol particles and triglycerides.

Wheat products spike blood sugar, yet the ADA still maintains that eating more grains is essential in a healthy diet.

Wheat contributes to the eventual death of pancreatic beta cells which control insulin response. Once we lose a certain percentage of these cells, diabetes is considered irreversible.

Wheat and grains are unique among plant-based foods in that they form acid in the body, contributing to inflammation and robbing bones of minerals.

Wheat contributes to the formation of AGEs, useless compounds which prematurely age virtually every part of the human body.

A diet free of wheat is not only healthy for the body, but may be considered an anti-aging diet as well.

Small LDL particles are a major risk factor for heart disease and stroke. Wheat products greatly increase small LDL particle levels in the blood.

Current testing methods are outdated. Seek out a doctor who will perform the latest and most accurate tests for a true picture of your small LDL levels (such as NMR lipoprotein analysis).

Fat actually does very little to affect overall triglyceride levels, while wheat products do a great deal.

Eliminating wheat products can reduce or eliminate a host of conditions which lead to chronic and life-threatening conditions, including many forms of heart disease.

Wheat can affect the brain in many ways, including decreased mental clarity, addictive behavior, seizures, ataxia and other neurological conditions, cell death and dementia.

A wide range of skin disorders respond well to wheat elimination, including many which commonly "require" the use of painful, costly and dangerous medications.

Wheat Belly: Section 3

Eliminating Wheat

Eliminating all wheat from your diet can seem scary and intimidating at first. After all, it's incredibly pervasive – nearly every meal and snack we consume contains wheat. Dr. Davis maintains that it can be done and once you make that initial break, the health benefits you'll enjoy will make you very happy you did.

It's important to remember that there is no potential for a "wheat deficiency." We don't need any wheat to survive. In fact, on average, we improve amazingly without wheat.

What you replace your wheat with is essential. If you cut out wheat but eat junk to fill the gap, you won't see many benefits. Instead, Dr. Davis recommends increasing your consumption of real, whole foods. These foods will not leave you feeling deprived, but will actually leave you more satisfied than if you had filled up on junk.

Fiber is a common worry, but an unfounded one. When you eliminate wheat, you will naturally eat more vegetables to fill the calorie gap. This will give you all the fiber you need.

How to Do It

While Dr. Davis explains that getting rid of wheat is the important part, how you do it can mean the difference between a clean break and agonizing relapses. Dr. Davis recommends ridding your life (and your kitchen) of wheat in one clean sweep. Wheat cravings disappear sometime around the third day of a wheat-free life. Once you get past this initial craving period, going wheat-free becomes much easier.

If you're worried that a wheat-free lifestyle will mean more work, don't despair. Dr. Davis maintains that once you're past the constant cycle of cravings created by wheat, eating becomes much simpler. You will eat because you are hungry, not because you are crazed with cravings. Your meals will keep you satisfied for longer periods of time. You will appreciate your food more. You may have to acquire some cooking skills and spend a bit more time at the supermarket, but the payoff is well worth the effort.

Fighting Through Withdrawals

Even if you don't think you're addicted to wheat, you may still experience an uncomfortable withdrawal period. Dr. Davis recommends scheduling this period (which typically lasts a few days) during time off from work or at least over a weekend. Dr. Davis states that wheat withdrawal is not dangerous, only annoying.

Dangers of Relapse

Once you've successfully gone wheat-free, Dr. Davis warns against what you might experience if you let yourself slide and have a serving of wheat. Even if you never before experienced adverse effects, putting wheat into your body after a period of wheat-free living can result in some nasty side effects, sometimes as severe as those of food poisoning. Proceed with caution.

Carbs to Consider Eliminating

Dr. Davis suggests that, as a society, we eat entirely too many carbohydrates. If you're really dedicated to improved health, he advises removing several other substances from your diet, or at least reducing their consumption. These include: cornmeal and cornstarch, snack foods, processed gluten-free foods, sugary desserts, rice, potatoes, sugary drinks, dried fruits and large servings of other grains including quinoa, buckwheat and oats.

Cured meats and anything with hydrogenated (trans) fats should also be eliminated from the diet.

What to Eat

You might be feeling a bit nervous right about now, wondering what you *can* eat. Don't despair – your options are wide, varied and delicious.

Load up on all vegetables. You may want to consult some vegetarian cookbooks or websites to remind yourself just how versatile vegetables can be.

Try some fruit, but don't overdo it – because of their high sugar content, almost all fruits are best in moderation only. Look for berries first, and restrict bananas, mangoes and pineapples.

Raw nuts make a wonderful snack and reduce LDL cholesterol levels. Dr. Davis asserts that you can't eat too many. Just make sure they're raw – stay away from any cooking processes which add fats or sugars. Peanuts shouldn't be eaten raw, so look for boiled or dry-roasted varieties with no additional ingredients.

Healthy oils are your friends. Use them generously. Olive oil is a familiar healthy oil, but coconut, avocado and even cocoa butter are all healthy alternatives.

Have a steak! Dr. Davis asserts that the meat and eggs we've "feared" for so long are actually just fine; it's only when their saturated fats are combined with carbohydrates that negative health effects can occur. Purchase grass-fed and organic whenever possible and listen to your body; it will tell you when it's hungry and what it wants.

Dr. Davis also makes the distinction that while cheese is a wonderful food to be enjoyed anytime you like, other dairy products, because of their ability to stimulate insulin production, should be restricted to once or twice per day.

Flaxseed is unique; it does not create the negative effects of other grains. Use it as often as you like. In addition, explore different condiments and spices to liven up your meals. Drink water in favor of other beverages. Soy products should be consumed only if they are not genetically modified, which can be difficult to determine.

The average person, according to Dr. Davis, does best by limiting carbohydrate intake to about 50 to 100 grams per day. Dr. Davis cautions that individual carbohydrate needs will vary. For example, if you're trying to reverse diabetes, a more rigid carb restriction should be enforced (perhaps 30 grams or less). Athletes require more carbs, so adjust carb intake while training or competing.

Once you've overcome the initial period of withdrawals, you'll likely experience a reduction in a wide variety of health issues, increased feelings of well-being and a heightened appreciation for your meals. Going wheat-free can be difficult, but the rewards are well worth the effort. Clear out your kitchen, stock up on real, whole foods and get ready to experience the amazing results of a wheat-free life!

Looking For More?

Shortcut Summaries strongly encourages you to buy and read the full version of Wheat Belly by William Davis MD for much more information on this topic. You'll also get all his interesting personal stories, the supporting studies he provides, plus his wheat-free menu ideas. You can find it at Amazon.com by performing this search:

Wheat Belly by William Davis MD: Lose the Wheat, Lose the Weight and Find Your Path Back to Health

Also, be sure to check out the Wheat Belly Cookbook by William Davis MD. Search using the text below to purchase from Amazon:

Wheat Belly Cookbook by William Davis MD: 150 Recipes to Help You Lose the Wheat, Lose the Weight, and Find Your Path Back to Health

Other Popular Best Selling Diet Books For Kindle and Print

We have listed both the short titles and the full titles of these books to make them easier to locate.

You can also search Amazon.com for "diet books best sellers 2012" or "diet books best sellers 2011" for an up to date listing.

Good Calories, Bad Calories by Gary Taubes

The Blood Sugar Solution by Mark Hyman

The Blood Sugar Solution: The UltraHealthy Program for Losing Weight, Preventing Disease, and Feeling Great Now! by Mark Hyman

Why We Get Fat by Gary Taubes

Why We Get Fat: And What to Do About It by Gary Taubes

The Art and Science of Low Carbohydrate Living by Stephen Phinney and Jeff Volek

The Art and Science of Low Carbohydrate Living: An Expert Guide to Making the Life-Saving Benefits of Carbohydrate Restriction Sustainable and Enjoyable by Stephen Phinney, Jeff Volek

The New Atkins for a New You by Dr. Eric C. Westman, Dr. Stephen D. Phinney, Jeff S. Volek

The Paleo Solution by Robb Wolf

The Paleo Solution: The Original Human Diet by Robb Wolf, or Rob Wolf

Wheat Belly by William Davis MD

Wheat Belly: Lose the Wheat, Lose the Weight, and Find Your Path Back To Health
by William Davis MD

The Primal Blueprint by Mark Sisson

The Primal Blueprint: Reprogram your genes for effortless weight loss, vibrant health and boundless energy by Mark Sisson

Forks Over Knives by Gene Stone

Forks Over Knives: The Plant-Based Way to Health by Gene Stone

Deadly Harvest by Geoff Bond

Deadly Harvest: The Intimate Relationship Between Our Heath and Our Food by Geoff Bond

The Rosedale Diet
by Ron Rosedale and Carol Colman

Ignore the awkward by Uffe Ravnskov

Ignore the awkward! How the cholesterol myths are kept alive by Uffe Ravnskov

Primal Body, Primal Mind by Nora Gedgaudas

Primal Body, Primal Mind: Beyond the Paleo Diet for Total Health and a Longer Life by Nora T. Gedgaudas, CNS, CNT

What to Eat by Marion Nestle

Deep Nutrition by Catherine Shanahan

Deep Nutrition: Why Your Genes Need Traditional Food by Catherine Shanahan MD

Weight Loss Books For Women, Teens or Men

You can also search for "weight loss books best sellers 2012" or "weight loss best sellers 2011" for a current list.

The Atkins Diet

Dr. Atkins' New Diet Revolution by Robert C. Atkins

The Skinny Rules by Bob Harper

The Skinny Rules: The Simple, Nonnegotiable Principles for Getting to Thin by Bob Harper

Protein Power by Dr. Eades

Protein Power: The High-Protein/Low-Carbohydrate Way to Lose Weight, Feel Fit, and Boost Your Health--in Just Weeks!
by Michael R. Eades, Mary Dan Eades

Eat to Live by Dr. Joel Fuhrman

Eat to Live: The Amazing Nutrient-Rich Program for Fast and Sustained Weight Loss by Joel Fuhrman

The Paleo Answer by Loren Cordain

The Paleo Answer: 7 Days to Lose Weight, Feel Great, Stay Young by Loren Cordain

The Seventeen Day Diet by Mike Moreno

The 17 Day Diet by Mike Moreno

The China Study by T. Colin Campbell

The China Study: The Most Comprehensive Study of Nutrition Ever Conducted And the Startling Implications for Diet by T. Colin Campbell

Choose to Lose by Chris Powell

Choose to Lose: The 7-Day Carb Cycle Solution by Chris Powell

Fit2Fat2Fit by Drew Manning

Fit2Fat2Fit: The Unexpected Lessons from Gaining and Losing 75 lbs on Purpose by Drew Manning

The Belly Fat Diet by John Chatham

The Belly Fat Diet: Lose Your Belly, Shed Excess Weight, Improve Health by John Chatham

The Dukan Diet Book by Pierre Dukan

The Dukan Diet: 2 Steps to Lose the Weight, 2 Steps to Keep It Off Forever by Pierre Dukan

The Mayo Clinic Diet Book

The Mayo Clinic Diet: Eat Well, Enjoy Life, Lose Weight by Mayo Clinic

The Mayo Clinic Diabetes Diet by Mayo Clinic

The Virgin Diet by JJ Virgin

The Virgin Diet: Drop 7 Foods, Lose 7 Pounds, Just 7 Days by JJ Virgin

101 Best Foods to Boost Your Metabolism by Metabolic-Calculator.com

Pure Fat Burning Fuel by Isabel De Los Rios

Pure Fat Burning Fuel: Follow This Simple, Heart Healthy Path To Total Fat Loss
by Isabel De Los Rios

It Starts with Food by Melissa Hartwig

It Starts with Food: Discover the Whole30 and

Change Your Life in Unexpected Ways
by Melissa Hartwig

The Four Hour Body by Timothy Ferriss

The 4-Hour Body: The Secrets and Science of Rapid
Body Transformation by Timothy Ferriss

Wheat Belly Cookbook by William Davis MD

Wheat Belly Cookbook: 150 Recipes to Help You
Lose the Wheat, Lose the Weight, and Find Your
Path Back to Health by William Davis MD

CPSIA information can be obtained at www.ICGtesting.com
Printed in the USA
LVOW101819200113

316455LV00022B/1203/P